If I Can't Eat Flies, What Am I?

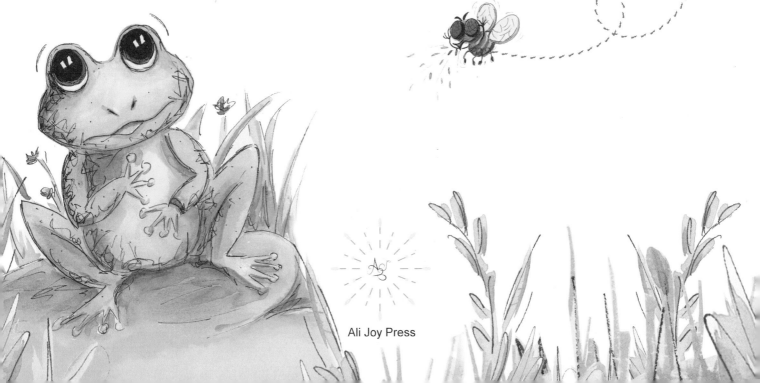

Ali Joy Press

Thank you to Gus, Belen, Melanie, Louie, Craig, and all my other friends and family who provided support, feedback, and inspiration; and, to Paula for your breathtaking ink and watercolor illustrations that made my story come to life! Cheers to checking off a bucket list item together.
~Alicia

Thank you to my family for their patience, understanding and support while I worked for countless hours to bring Tad and his friends to life, and to Alicia for giving me the opportunity to illustrate your beautiful story.
~Paula

If I Can't Eat Flies, What Am I?

Text copyright © 2021 Alicia J. Pfaff
Cover art and interior illustrations copyright © 2021 Paula M. Zelienka

Edited by Jennifer Rees
Cover & book design by Stephanie Drake

Learn more!
www.aliciajpfaff.com

ISBN 978-1-7359899-0-7 (hardcover) | ISBN 978-1-7359899-1-4 (softcover) | ISBN 978-1-7359899-4-5 (ebook)

Library of Congress Control Number: 2020924815

First Edition

Ali Joy Press
PO Box 88
Palmerton, PA 18071

To Logan, who has lived his childhood with multiple severe allergies and was the inspiration for this book—and all other children with food allergies who struggle with feeling different at a time in your life when you so desperately want to fit in, and with learning at far too young of an age that you are not competely invincible.

—A.J.P.

To Jesse, our very picky little book critic who let me know I painted the right Tad by breaking out in a huge smile, hugging Tad's painting, and carrying it around the house; and, to Maddie, who was there every step of the way to listen to my ideas, share her thoughts, and lend a hand whenever needed. I couldn't have done it without you.

—P.M.Z.

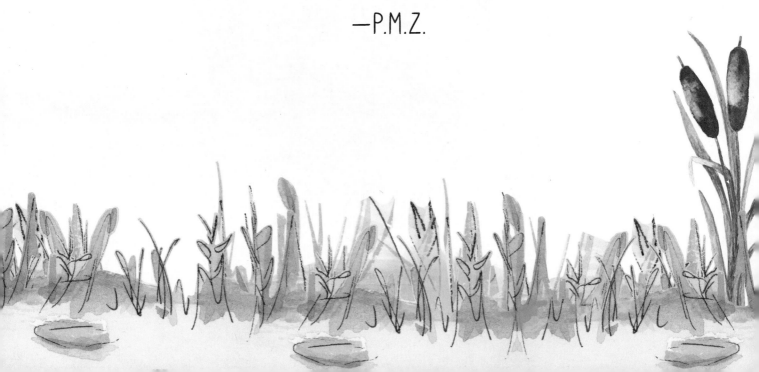

Hello. My name is Tad. I'm a frog, or so I thought.
I'm feeling really sad because the doctor says I've got—

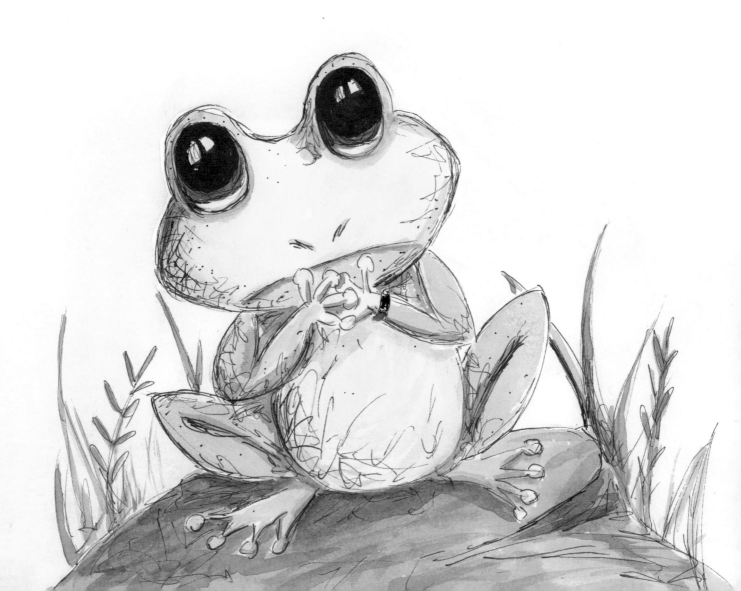

a food allergy—to **flies!**
They make me really sick.
My allergy is so bad, I can't even risk a lick.

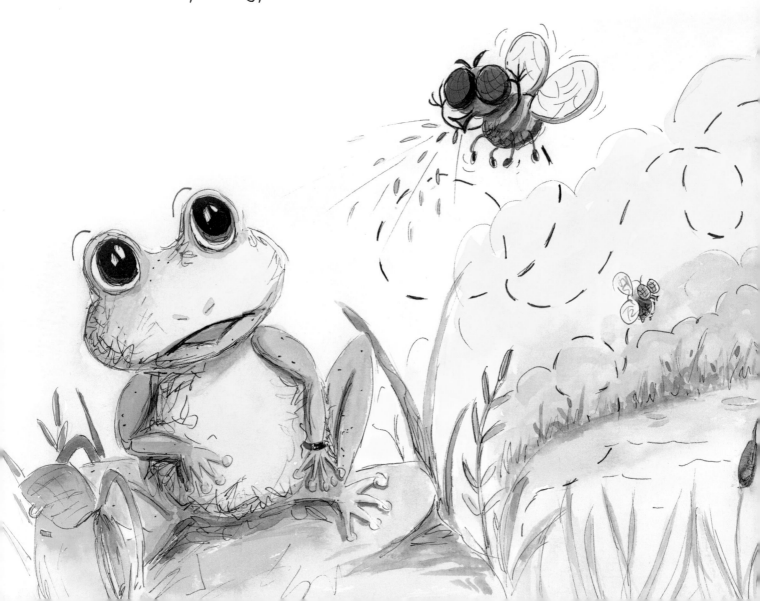

I'd love to eat those yummy flies,
but then I would break out in hives.
Hives itch, **a lot!**
It would get hard for me to breathe,
and I'd have to get a shot.

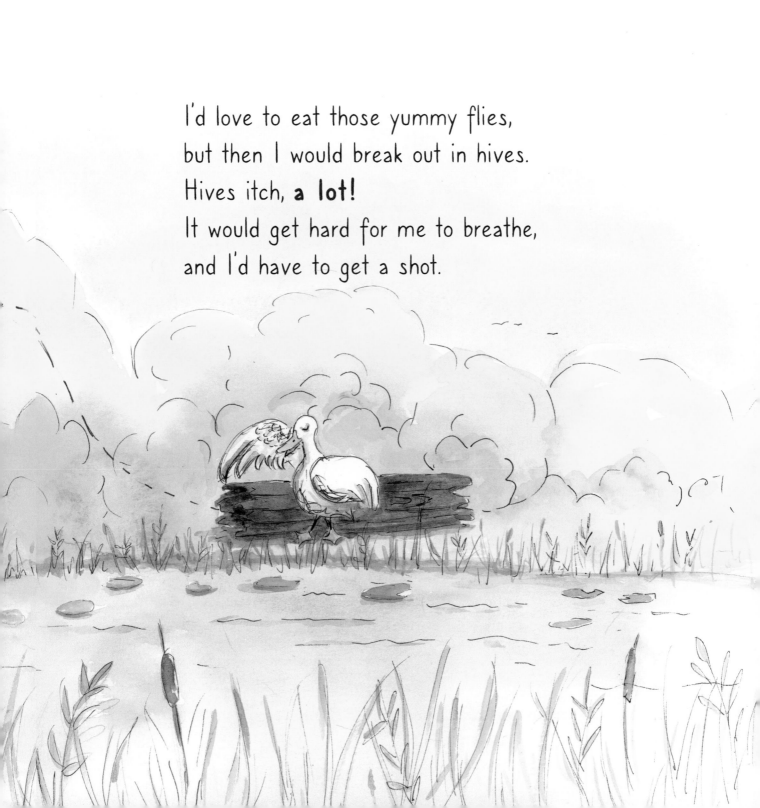

I'm just so different from my friends and family.
I don't think I'm a frog; it's very obvious to me.

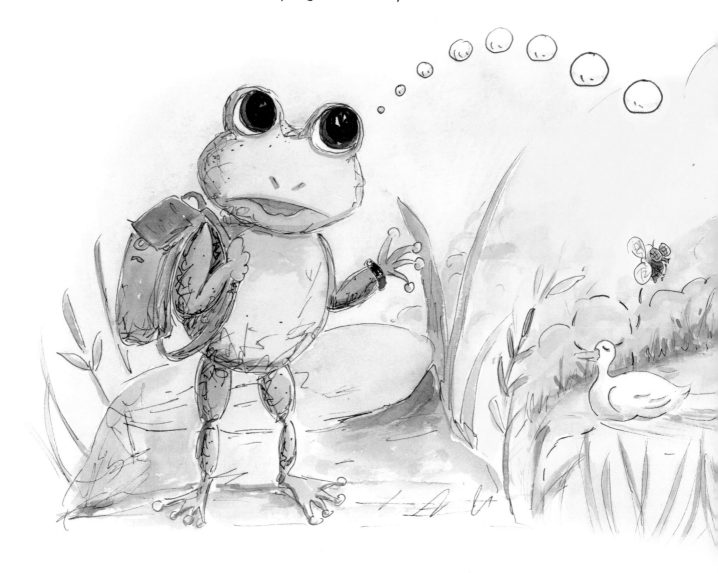

So, I'm going on a journey to see what I might be.

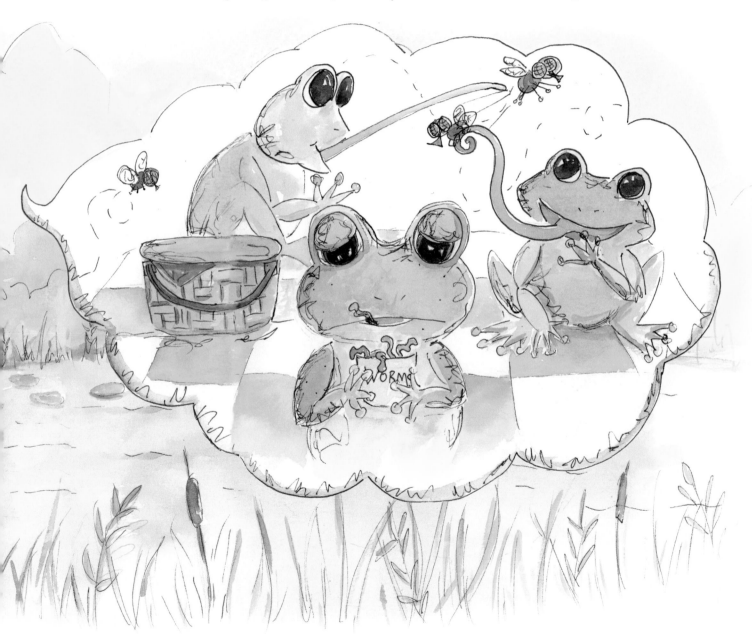

"Hello, my name is Tad. I'm glad we get to meet!
I'm wondering if you'd tell me what ducks like to eat?"

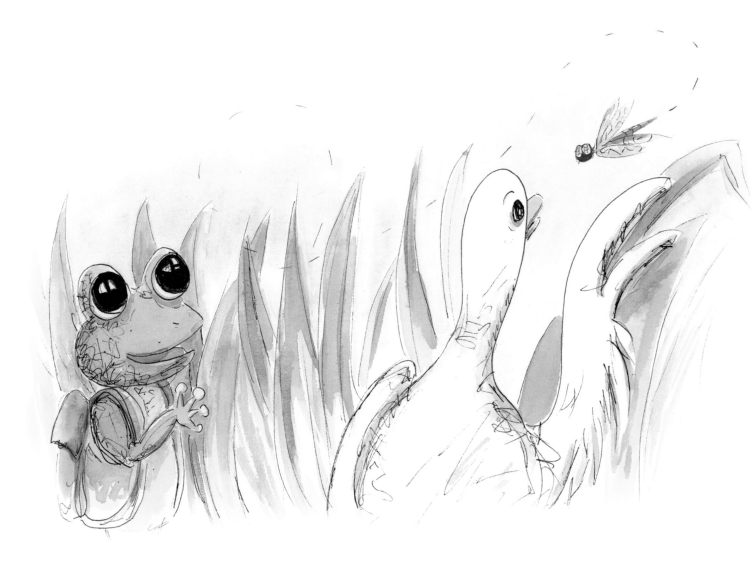

"Shhh! I'm Mia, and I'm hoping to eat that dragonfly, right there, as a very special treat."

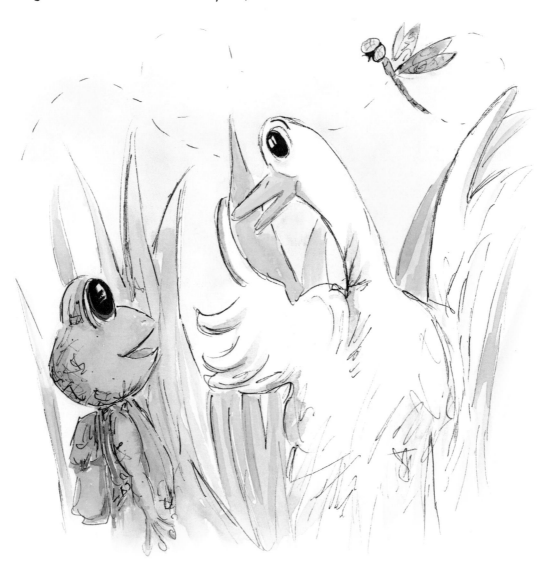

"Oooh, I like dragonflies," Tad says. "Maybe I can help!"

Wah-Peesh!

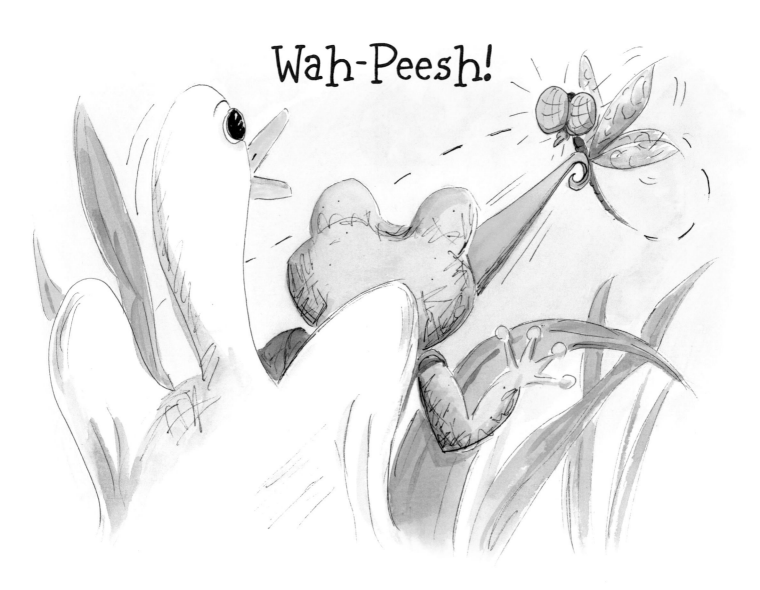

"No way!" Mia cries. "You can have it now.

Sheesh!"

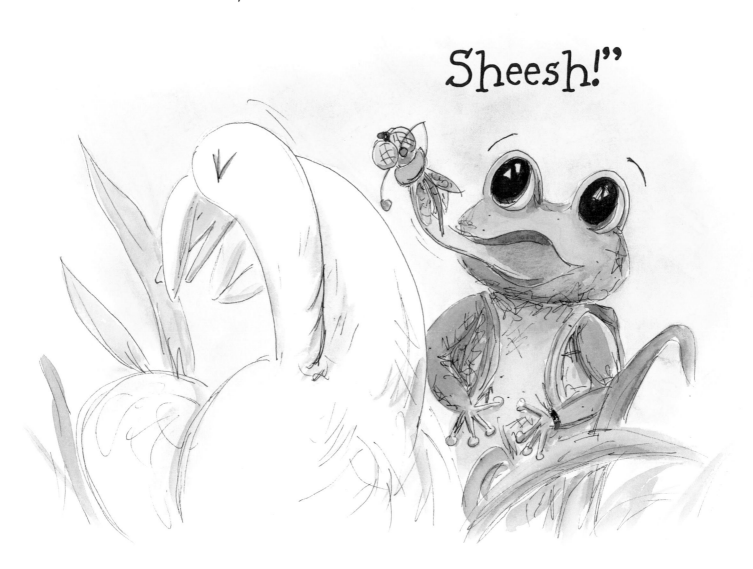

"Hey! Maybe I'm a duck! We both eat dragonflies."

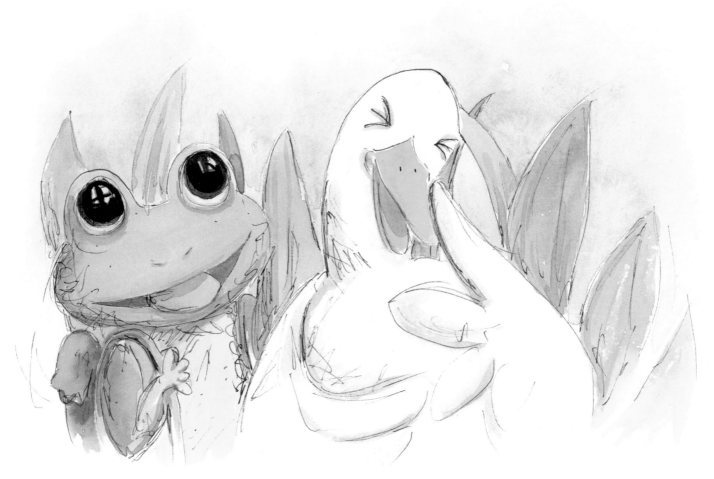

"Silly Frog," Mia says, "you can't even fly!
Go ahead, I double-duck-dare you to try."

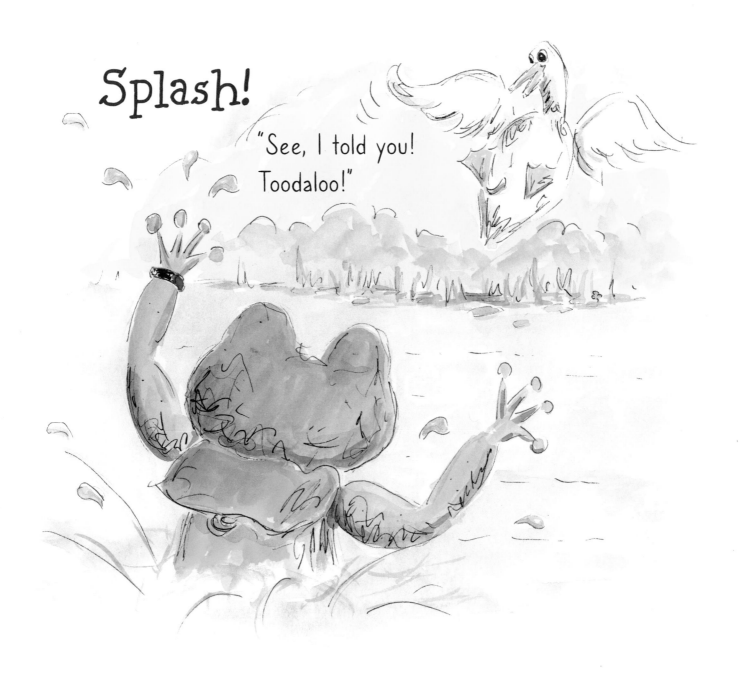

"Hi, there," Tad says, "I'm sorry I intruded.
May I ask what you're doing?
And, may I be included?"

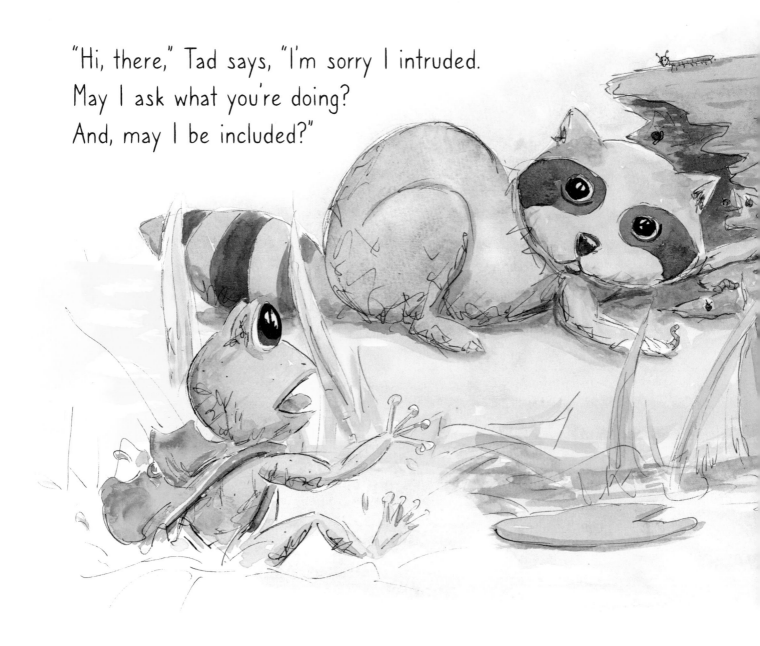

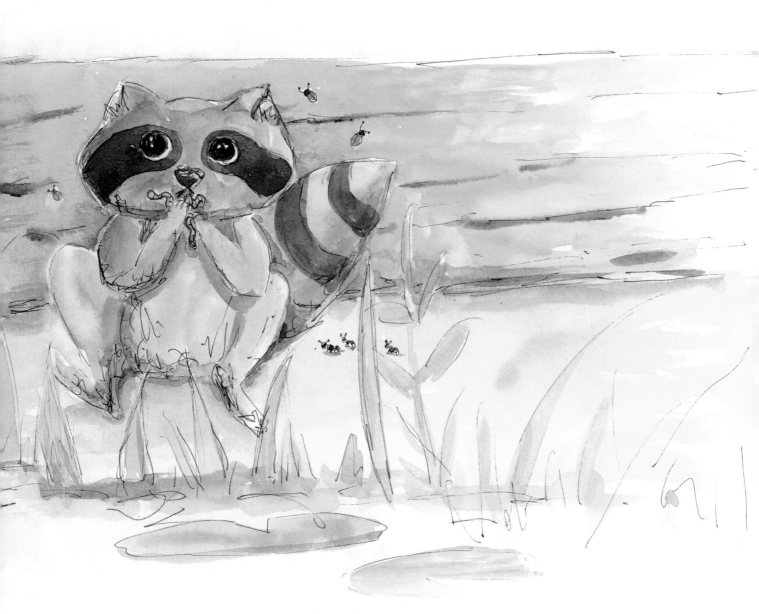

"Hi," Rax says. "You're an odd little frog!
Rocco and I are eating bugs from this log."

"You're wrong! I'm **NOT** a frog
because I can't eat flies;
but, I'm able to eat these bugs.
Can I be a raccoon like you guys?"

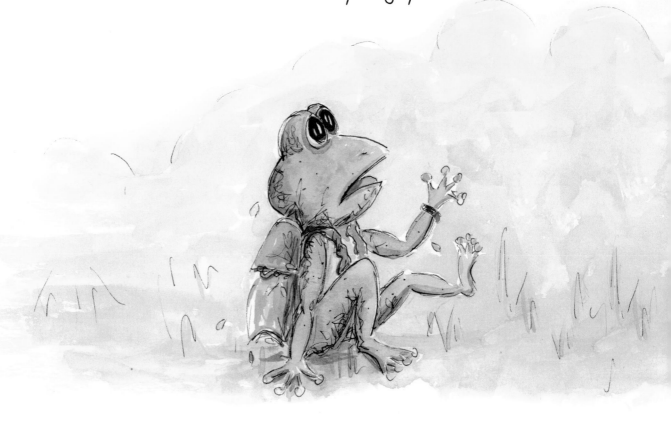

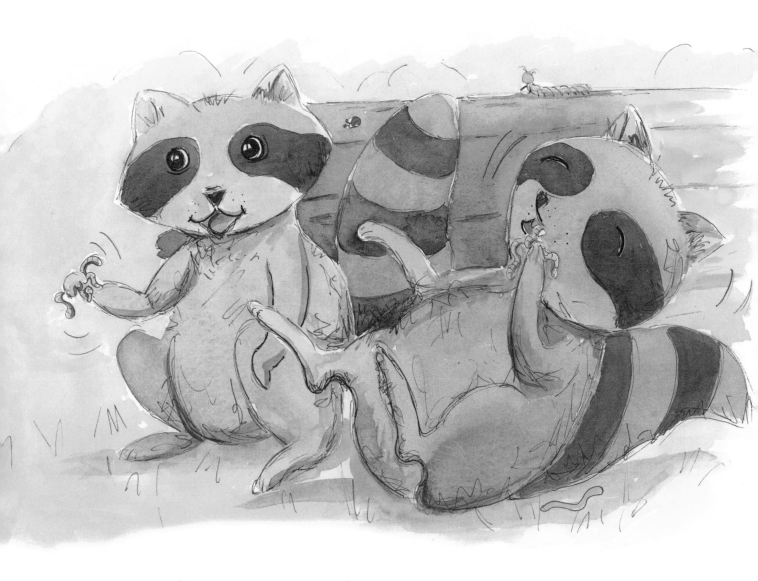

"Silly frog, you can't be a raccoon!
Mamma eats frogs, and she'll be back soon."

Tad runs away—**fast**—looking back in fear.

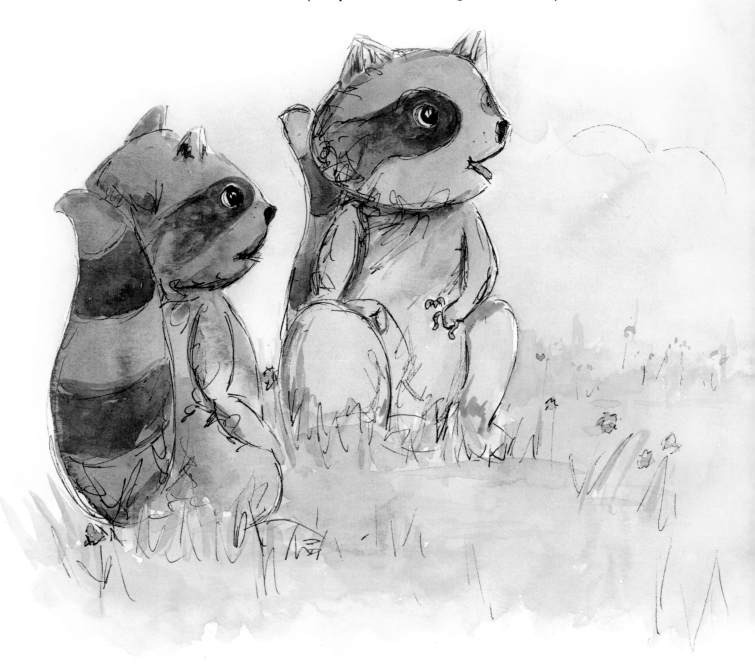

He doesn't realize that
Cara the cow is very near.

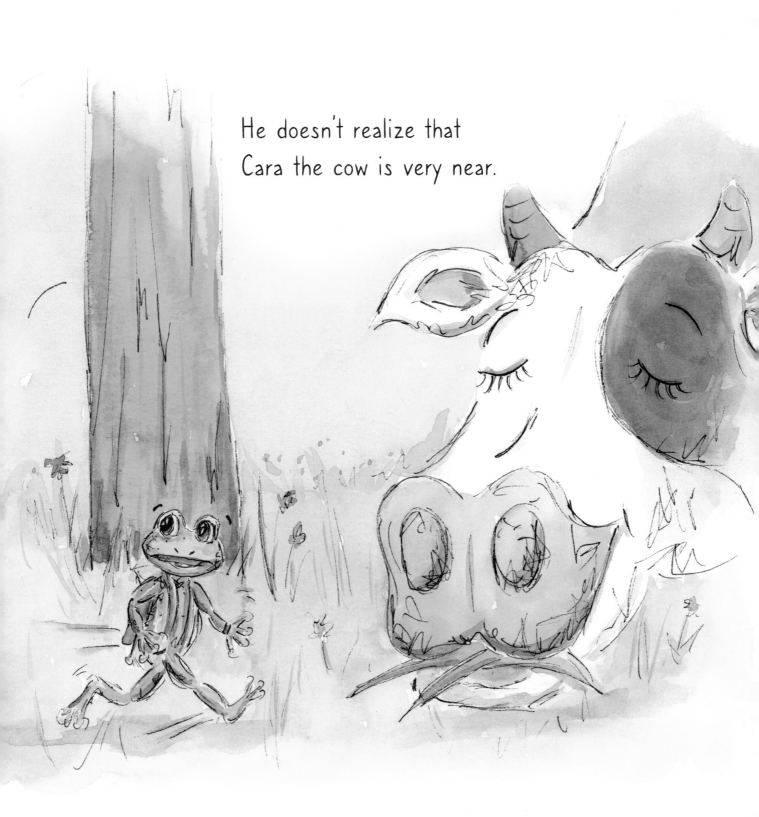

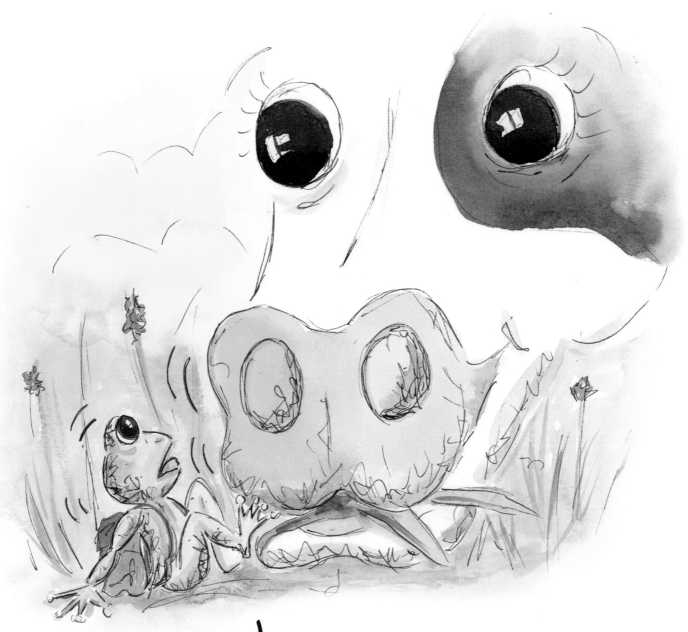

Whump!

Cara chuckles. "Hello, little Tad.
Why are you out and about?"

"It seems I'm not a frog.
But, what am I? I need to find out."

"Why do you think you are not a frog?
You are green with buggy eyes.
You certainly look like a frog,
and, you know, Miss Cara is very wise"

"Then, you must know that **all** frogs eat flies.
But, if I eat flies, I break out in hives!
So, I can't be a frog. Don't you see?
A frog is something I must not be."

"Hmm, you say eating flies makes you break out in hives? Maybe the problem is that you can't eat **live** flies.

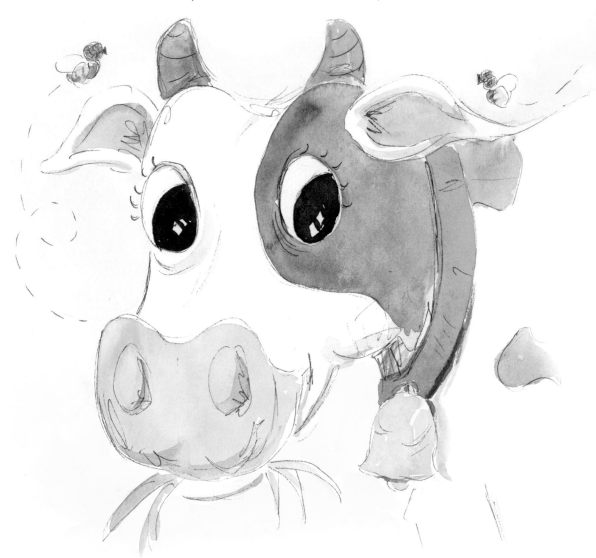

My famous moo-fly pie is truly delish and is made
with **dead** flies I swat with my tail—

swish,
swish!"

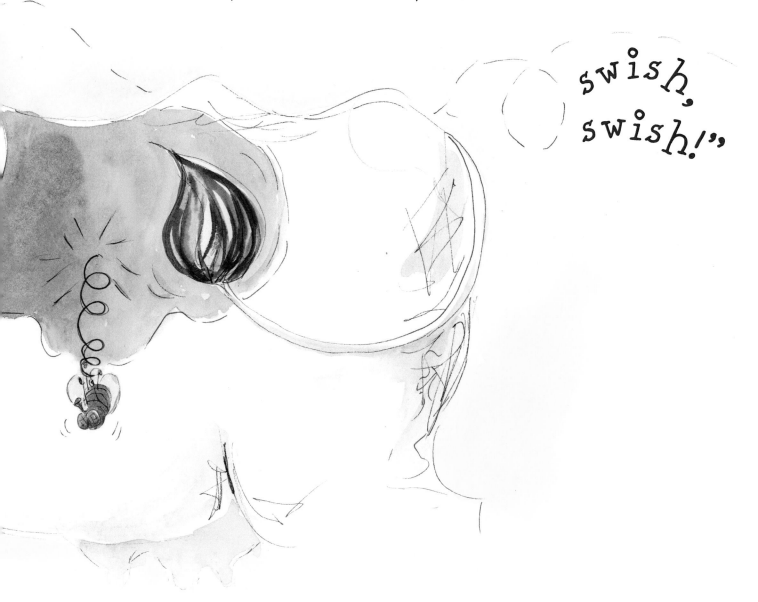

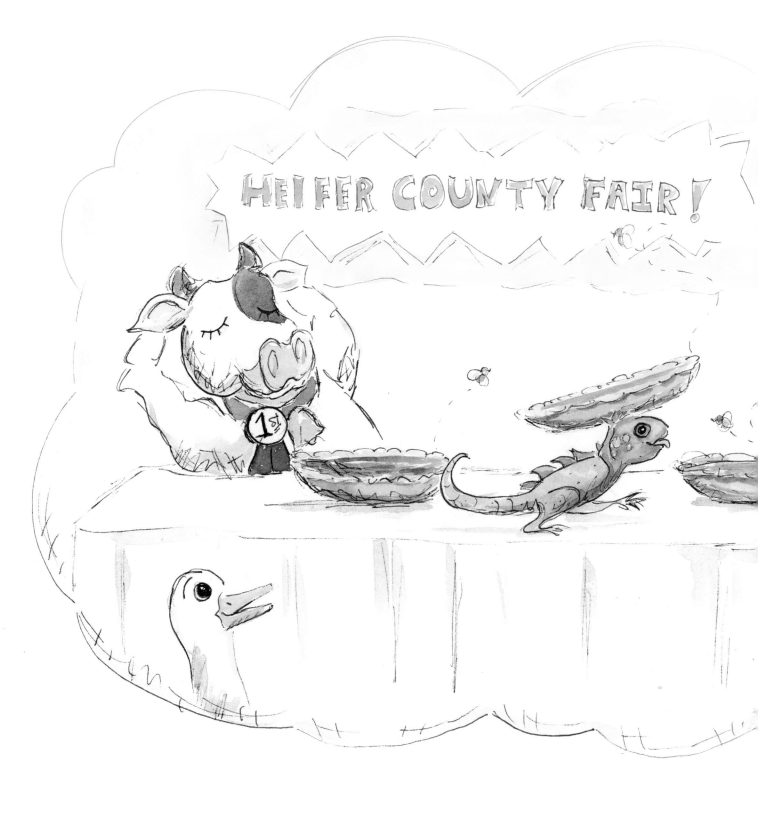

"It wins first prize at the Heifer County fair,
though it doesn't last long once the iguanas get there."

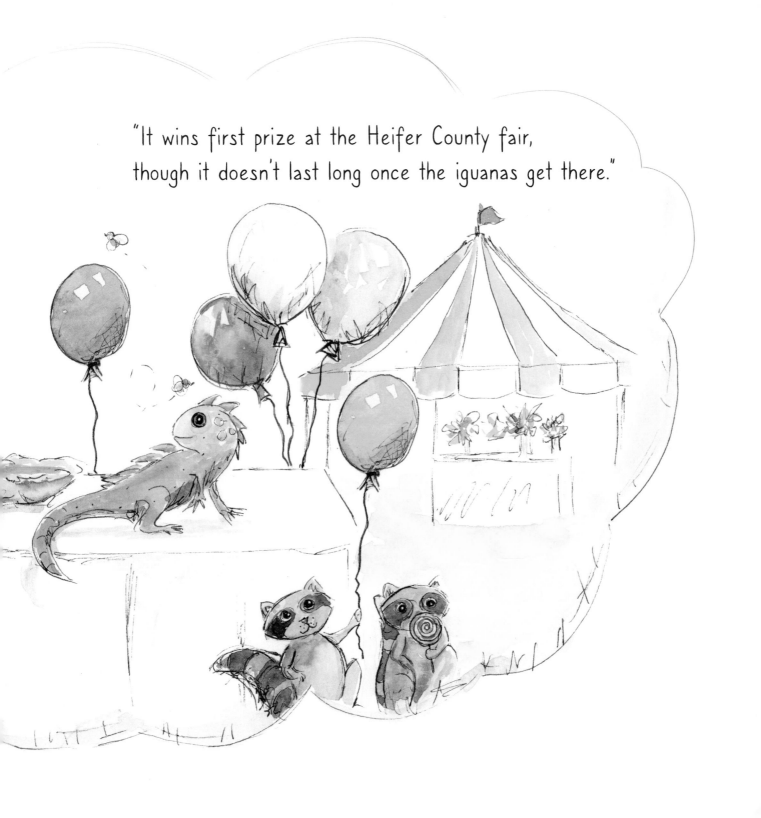

"I think dead or alive, in a pie, or on a log,
a fly is a fly; and you would still be a frog!"

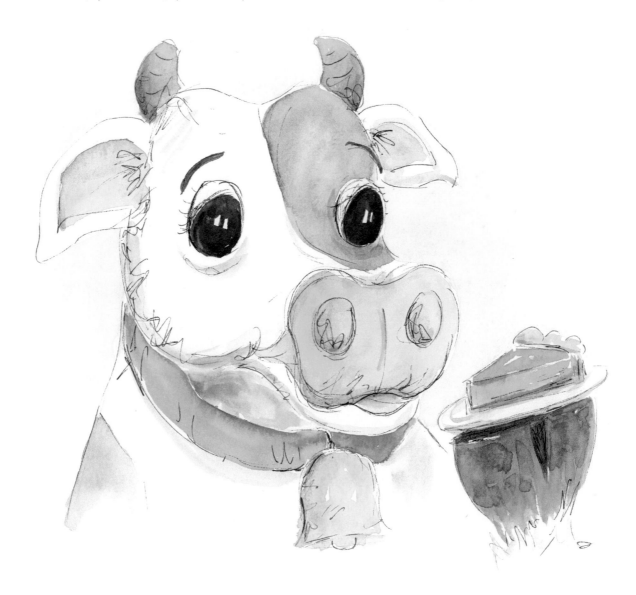

"I'm so excited, I think you may be right!
Let me try your pie, please!
I'll just take a small bite."

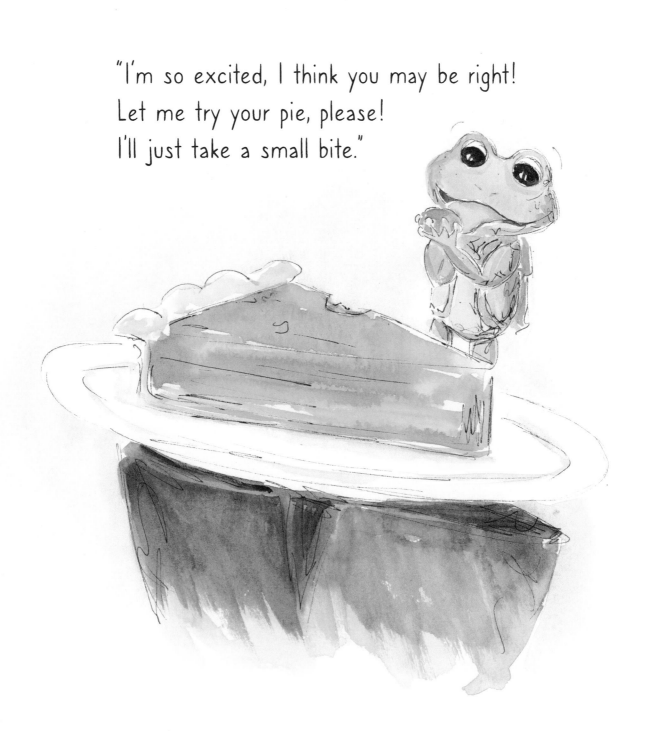

"Oh, no! Here come the hives, and my chest feels tight.
HELP! Call 9-1-1! I am definitely not alright!"

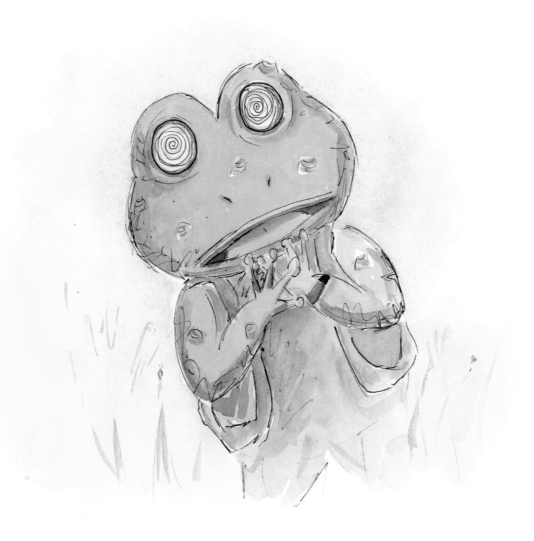

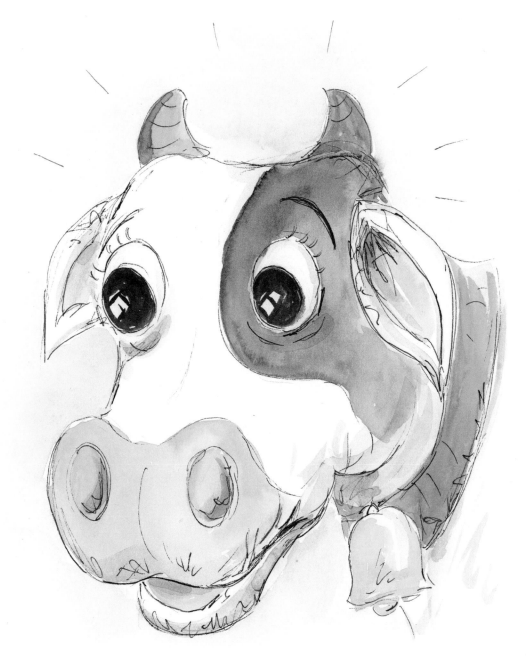

"Don't worry, Tad," Cara says. "I called the Medic Bees. They will be here soon. Won't you forgive me, please?"

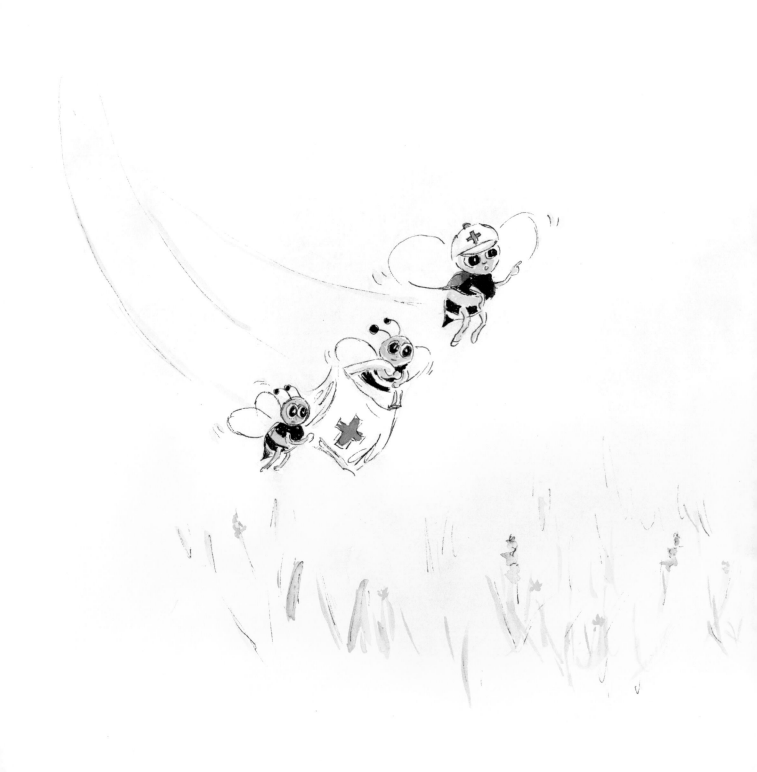

"It's okay," Tad whispers. "You were trying to help me. Now we know, dead flies are not safe—**no siree!**"

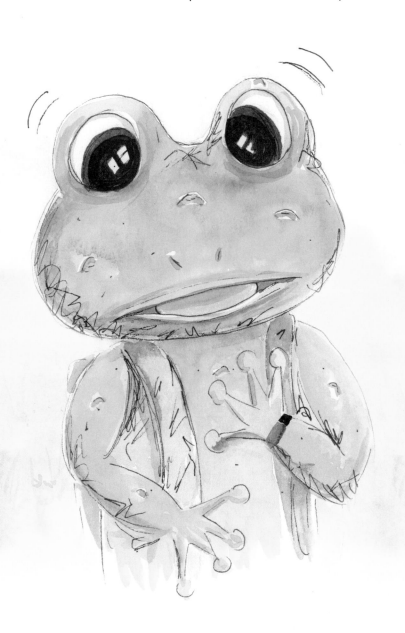

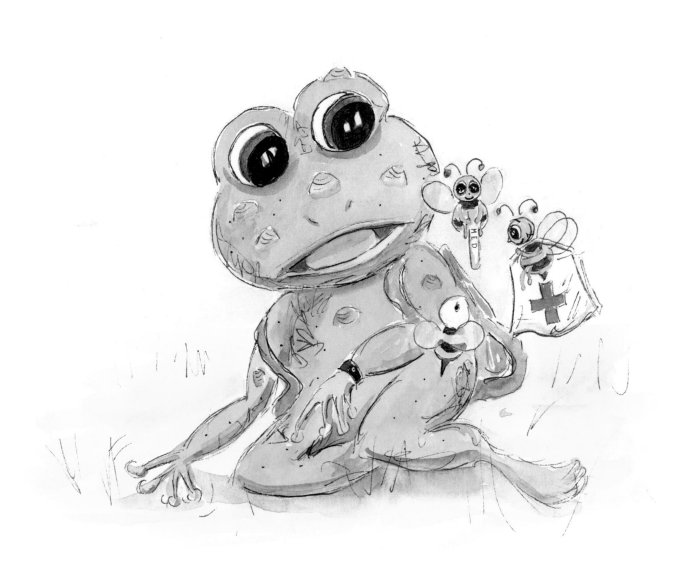

Medic arrives and his team prepares Tad's shot.
Then, Medic uses his stinger in just the right spot.

"Tad," Medic says, "you know you can't eat flies.
So, trying moo-fly-pie was not very wise."

"I really am sorry," Tad explains. "I just want to belong.
A frog who can't eat flies—it just feels so wrong."

"Being different can be hard,
but, you'll figure it out somehow.
Someday, you may find it's a gift,
even if you don't think so right now."

"How would you know?" Tad's eyes fill with tears.

"Because, I'm allergic to honey—have been for years!
Since I couldn't make honey like other bees do,
I trained as a Medic, and now I get to help you!"

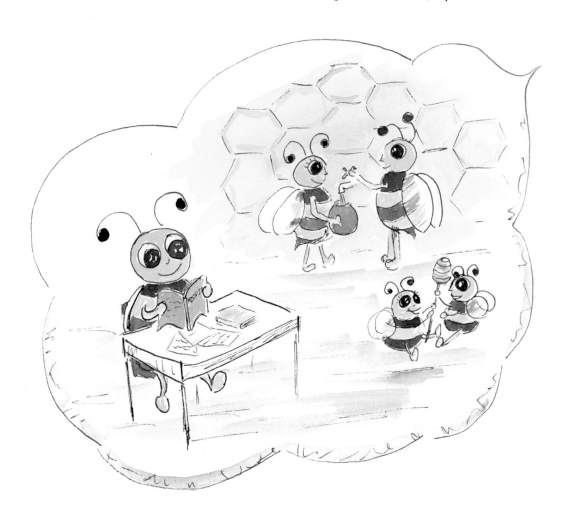

"Instead of focusing on what you cannot do, be thankful for what you **can**. Always carry your medicine with you, and don't ever eat flies again.

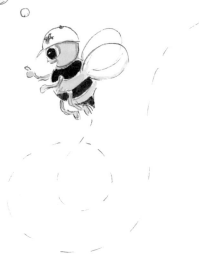

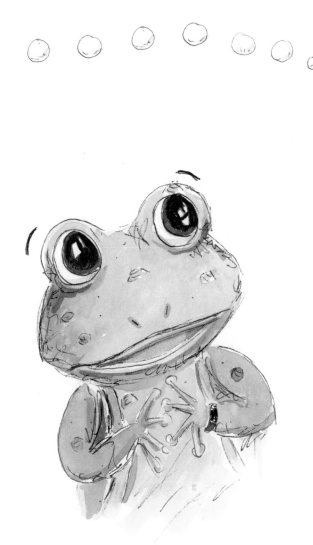

Oh, and never try a new food unless your parents say it's safe, because others, like Miss Cara, don't understand and may make mistakes."

"Look, here come your parents! They were worried about you.

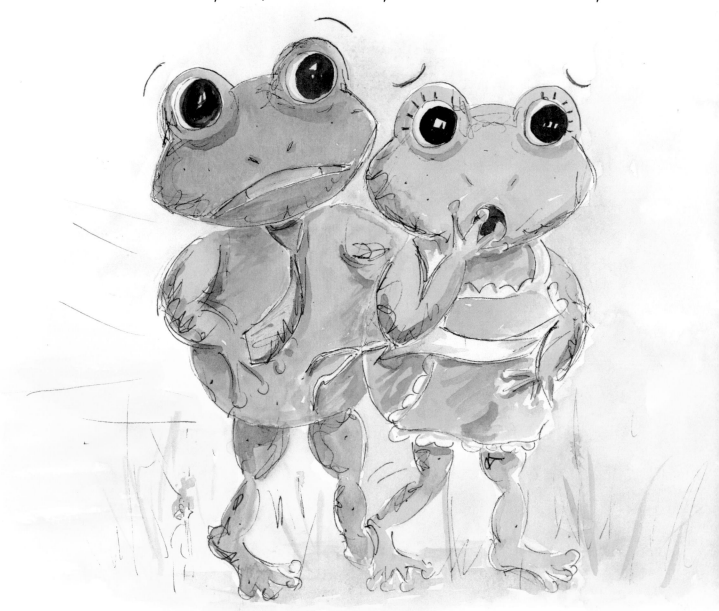

Remember, you are very special, even if you can't eat what others do: that includes live flies, dead flies, or flies cooked in a stew."

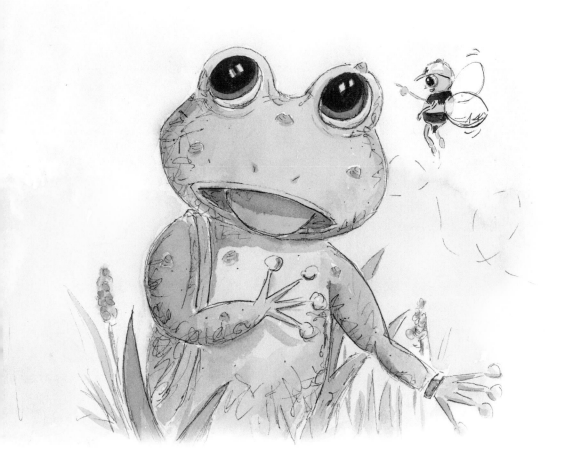

"Mom! Dad! I'm sorry I scared you guys.
I guess to be a frog, I don't have to eat flies."
His parents hug him with all of their might.

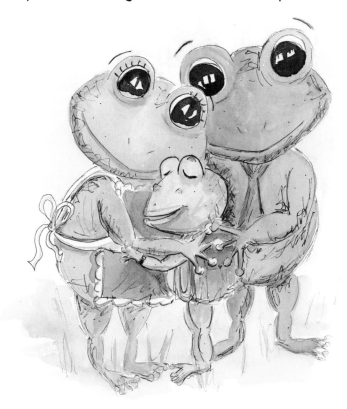

"That's correct, Taddy Bear. We're so glad you're all right!
It's not what you eat, but what's here, inside, that defines
who you are and fills us with pride!"

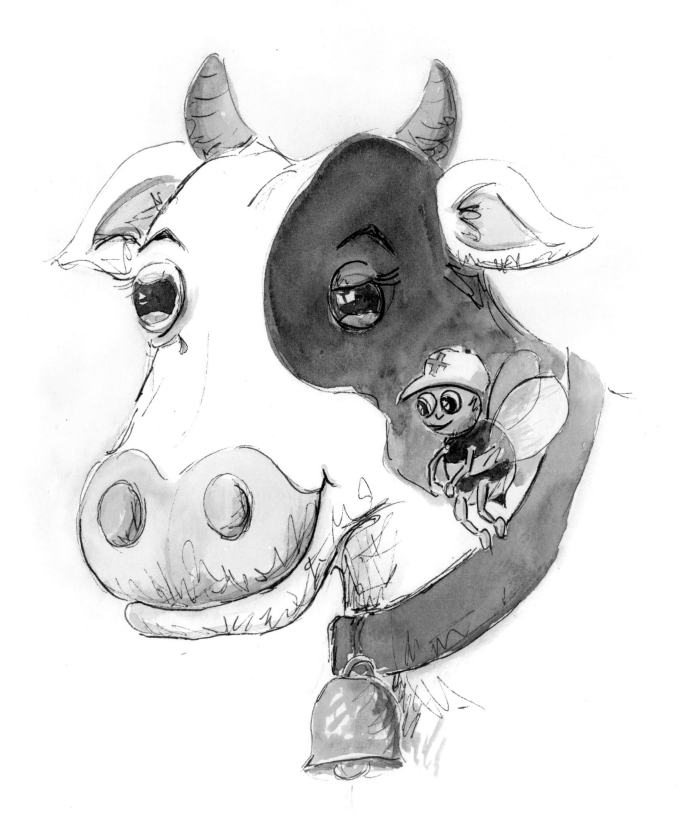

Hello, again! I came for a checkup, since Medic gave me that shot. Look how many friends and family showed up! They all care, whether I eat flies or not.

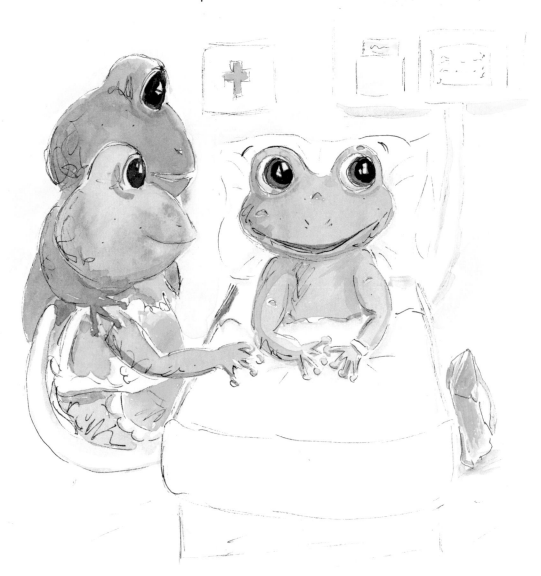

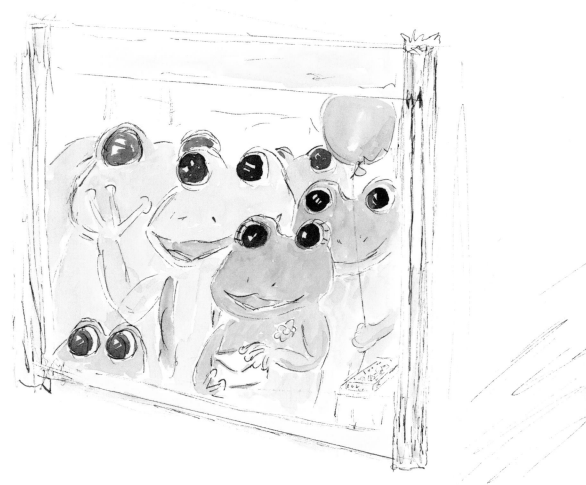

There are a lot of fabulous foods I **can** eat,
so, the answer I finally realize!

If I can't eat flies, what am I?

I'm still a fantastic frog—who just happens to **not** eat flies.

CPSIA information can be obtained
at www.ICGtesting.com
Printed in the USA
LVRC010729100421
683867LV00012B/110